Jodat Askari
Nazia Yazdanie

Acrylic Resins in Dentistry

Jodat Askari
Nazia Yazdanie

Acrylic Resins in Dentistry

LAP LAMBERT Academic Publishing

Impressum / Imprint
Bibliografische Information der Deutschen Nationalbibliothek: Die Deutsche Nationalbibliothek verzeichnet diese Publikation in der Deutschen Nationalbibliografie; detaillierte bibliografische Daten sind im Internet über http://dnb.d-nb.de abrufbar.
Alle in diesem Buch genannten Marken und Produktnamen unterliegen warenzeichen-, marken- oder patentrechtlichem Schutz bzw. sind Warenzeichen oder eingetragene Warenzeichen der jeweiligen Inhaber. Die Wiedergabe von Marken, Produktnamen, Gebrauchsnamen, Handelsnamen, Warenbezeichnungen u.s.w. in diesem Werk berechtigt auch ohne besondere Kennzeichnung nicht zu der Annahme, dass solche Namen im Sinne der Warenzeichen- und Markenschutzgesetzgebung als frei zu betrachten wären und daher von jedermann benutzt werden dürften.

Bibliographic information published by the Deutsche Nationalbibliothek: The Deutsche Nationalbibliothek lists this publication in the Deutsche Nationalbibliografie; detailed bibliographic data are available in the Internet at http://dnb.d-nb.de.
Any brand names and product names mentioned in this book are subject to trademark, brand or patent protection and are trademarks or registered trademarks of their respective holders. The use of brand names, product names, common names, trade names, product descriptions etc. even without a particular marking in this work is in no way to be construed to mean that such names may be regarded as unrestricted in respect of trademark and brand protection legislation and could thus be used by anyone.

Coverbild / Cover image: www.ingimage.com

Verlag / Publisher:
LAP LAMBERT Academic Publishing
ist ein Imprint der / is a trademark of
OmniScriptum GmbH & Co. KG
Bahnhofstraße 28, 66111 Saarbrücken, Deutschland / Germany
Email: info@omniscriptum.com

Herstellung: siehe letzte Seite /
Printed at: see last page
ISBN: 978-3-659-38709-8

Zugl. / Approved by: lahore,de'montmorency college PCSIR Lahore,2004

Copyright © Jodat Askari, Nazia Yazdanie
Copyright © 2013 OmniScriptum GmbH & Co. KG
Alle Rechte vorbehalten. / All rights reserved. Saarbrücken 2013

CONTENTS

s.no	page no.
List of Figures	2
List of Tables	3
List of Abbreviations	4
1. Summary	5
2. Introduction	7
3. Purpose of study	11
4. Review of Literature	12
5. Material and Methods	31
6. Results	39
7. Discussion	51
8. Conclusion	59
9. References	63
10. Annexure	67

List of figures

Serial No.	Page No.
1: Reference points on teeth measuring the horizontal and anterio posterior movement of teeth	61
2: Reference line and occlusal reference points for measuring upward and downward movement of teeth.	61
3: Anatomical configuration of Maxillary cast	62
4: Posterior anchorage in Vig's Technique	62

List of tables

Serial No.	Page No.
Table 1 (a)	42
Table 1(b)	43
Table 1(c)	44
Table 2(a)	45
Table 2(b)	46
Table 2(c)	47
Table 3(a)	48
Table 3(b)	49
Table 3 (c)	50

List of Abbreviations.

MMA	Methylmethacrylate
diMMA	Dimethylmethacrylate
PMMA	Polymethylmethacrylate
0^c	degree centigrade.
%	percent
STD.	Standard deviation.
P	probabality variable
<	Less than
>	Greater than

SUMMARY:

Dimensional changes during processing of maxillary denture base leads to the movement of prosthetic teeth. The resultant occlusal disharmony poses problem for patient as well as for dentist, such as unstable denture, trauma to denture bearing tissues. Modifications and adjustments are made to achieve harmonious occlusion, which is time consuming.

The objective of this study was to compare three-dimensional movement of prosthetic teeth in Maxillary denture base using Conventional and Vig's processing techniques.

Ten Maxillary dentures were processed and divided into two groups of five each, Group A and Group B. They were processed by VIG'S and Conventional techniques. Amalgam fillings were placed in the buccal cusps of posterior, mid of incisal edges of anterior maxillary teeth. A reference line was engraved on the right and left sides of the cast. Three-dimensional movements of teeth were measured by measuring the distance between the reference line and cusp of teeth, between the cusps of posterior and anterior and anterior to anterior teeth, and between the teeth of the opposite segment of the arch, both manually and with a Transparency template for all respected reference points. The measuring procedure was repeated before and after processing of the maxillary denture.

CONCLUSION:

It is concluded from this study that Vig's method produced less movement in prosthetic teeth as compared to Conventional curing method at $p \geq 0.05$.

Therefore, it is recommended that to minimize occlusal disharmony in the complete dentures, Vig's processing technique should be employed for better post curing results.

INTRODUCTION:

Before the introduction of Acrylic resins Vulcanite was the most widely used denture base material. This was a highly cross-linked natural rubber that was difficult to process and pigment and become unhygienic due to salivary uptake.

Since mid 1940's [1-3, 17] denture bases have been fabricated using acrylic reins. These are resilient plastics formed by joining multiple Methylmethacrylate (MMA) molecules. Pure Acrylic (Polymethylmethacrylate (PMMA) is a colourless transparent solid but for dental use it can be tinted to provide almost any shade matching the oral tissues and degree of translucency. Though acrylic resin has many advantages such as easy processing / curing, but has a limitation of final contraction during curing. Dentist and students have been aware of this shrinkage which is 5% to 7% and is well documented in the literature.[1-19] This movement of teeth results in disturbed occlusion causing unstable dentures[4-7] causing trauma to the underlying denture bearing area. At the time of insertion, adjustment of denture base and occlusion causes wastage of time, loss of confidence on the part of patient and the dentist.

The movement of teeth may occur as a result of processing procedures and dimensional changes of acrylic denture base during curing, deflasking, finishing and polishing.

There is a consistent change in posterior teeth relationship before and after curing [1-5]. This problem arises due to the movement of maxillary posterior teeth in anterior direction in relation to mandibular posterior teeth. This can always be noted in cusped teeth after remounting the finished dentures which was different in the wax up stage. This movement changes the occlusion as it was in wax up stage.

An observation [3,4] revealed that the movement occurred only in maxillary denture. When a maxillary denture is first inserted in patient's mouth, disclosing paste demonstrate a derangement of rugae pattern, excessive contact in anterior palatal area and heavy contact of denture against the posterior slopes of tuberosities. This indicates the shrinkage occurring in forward direction in the maxillary denture base where as no such movement occur in mandibular denture base.

The reason is that in each instance the labial position of the maxillary alveolar ridge anchored the anterior part of the polymerizing and shrinking resin, thus all volumetric and linear contraction occurs in posterior region that causes the movement of teeth in forward direction [4,5].

This discrepancy of deranged occlusion at wax up stage and after curing has been solved by various methods, including advancement of denture base materials and different processing techniques [1-19].

Robert G Vig [3,4] studied this "polymerization shrinkage" mystery. He confirmed that this shrinkage was restricted to only maxillary denture base. In order to confirm his observations he used pins and metal jigs instead of teeth then cured the bases. The results were not different as he found previously. In order to over come the "problem of shrinkage" he gave a double thickness flap of wax over the posterior aspect of maxillary cast. This flap acted as an anchorage as alveolus in labial (anterior) aspect of maxilla.

He incorporated the pins and metal jigs, cured the bases with them. Amazingly no movement was found, the jigs were interdigitating exactly as in the wax up stage. Then he placed the teeth and repeated the whole procedure, and found that no movement had occurred.

Therefore the aim of this study is to compare two curing techniques i.e. Vig's and Conventional, in order to assess any significant movement in the maxillary denture base.

PURPOSE OF THE STUDY:

AIM:

The aim of this study is to compare two curing techniques i.e. Vig's and Conventional, in order to assess significantly less movement in the maxillary denture base.

OBJECTIVE:

To compare the 3-Dimensional movement of prosthetic teeth in maxillary complete denture base using Vig's and Conventional curing techniques.

LITERATURE REVIEW:

HISTORY OF ACRYLICS:

Centuries ago dentures were made of naturally occurring materials like hardwood, ivory, bone and natural the teeth held in these dentures bases by screws and plates [1-3, 17]

In 1851, Nelson Goodyear [17] developed a hard rubber named Vulcanite the use of which became very popular. This material besides its easy availability had some disadvantages as it was a highly cross linked rubber. It was difficult to process and technique sensitive, difficult to pigment and tended unhygienic due to salivary uptake. These short comings in Vulcanite made denturists to look for a newer, better and easy handling materials.

Advent of acrylic revolutionized the field of denture making. Acrylic acid and derivatives were well known even before 1890s, but in 1901 Dr.Otto Rhom [17] produced solid transparent polymers of acrylic acid. Derivatives of acrylic monomer i.e. methyl and ethyl acrylate were transparent liquids, highly volatile in nature. They were polymerized to give perfectly clear solid polymers. Initially developed polymers like acryloid, plexigum etc. were used for denture construction but they were not popularized due to their difficult fabrication, requiring expensive and complex equipment.

Phenol formaldehyde products were the first to compete with Vulcanite. These products were available in sheet cake and powder forms. However, the physical properties of final denture base depended heavily on the processing technique. By 1932 mixtures of Poly Vinyl Chloride (PVC) and Vinyl Acetate were available for use as denture base materials, but the associated processing technique resulted in high residual stresses. The base material often fractured shortly after insertion.

With the introduction of Veronite, Poly Methyl Methacrylate heat processed material, Vulcanite was discarded. Success of PMMA as a denture base, and its use as a definitive restorative material was attempted as well. By 1940 Veronite was being used for inlays, crowns and fixed partial dentures. After the

World War II the room temperature polymerization acrylic resins were made available in dentistry.

COMPOSITION OF ACRYLIC:

Acrylic resins are resilient plastics formed by joining Multiple Methyl MethAcrylate (MMA) molecules. Pure Poly Methyl MethAcrylate (PMMA) is a colourless transparent solid. It is supplied as powder liquid system.

Powder:

Major component of powder is beads of polymethylmethacrylate. These are produced by a process called "suspension polymerization" in which MMA monomer, containing initiator is suspended in water as droplets. Starch or Carboxy Methylcellulose can be used as thickeners and suspension stabilizers. The temperature is raised in order to decompose peroxide and bring about polymerization of MMA to form beads of PMMA, which after drying form free flowing powder at room temperature.

Initiator present in powder may consist of peroxide remaining unreacted after production of beads, in addition to extra peroxide added to beads after manufacture. Pink pigments used in denture base resins are traditionally salts of Cadmium.

Liquid:

Major component of liquid is MMA monomer. It is a colourless, low viscosity with a boiling point of $100.8°$ C. Ethylene Glycol Methylmethacrylate is added as cross linking agent, and Hydroquinone as an inhibitor.

TYPES OF ACRYLIC RESINS:

According to mode of polymerization acrylics can be classified as:

i) Heat curing

ii) Self / cold curing.

iii) Light curing.

MODE OF HEAT CURING:

The heat curing acrylic resins may be cured in one of the following ways:

1) Hot water bath:

The heating process used to control polymerization is termed as polymerization cycle.

Various cycles for curing of Acrylic denture base are used.

a. Long curing cycle:

b. Intermediate curing cycle:

c. Short curing cycle:

a) Long curing cycle:

In this curing cycle the denture base is in a constant water bath at 74°C for eight hours with no terminal bathing.

b) Intermediate curing cycle:

This curing cycle involves processing of denture base at $74°C$ for two hours then increasing the temperature of the water bath to $100°C$ and processing for another one hour more.

c) Short curing cycle:

The flask containing the acrylic dough is placed into boiling water, exothermic heat of reaction can cause the dough to reach a temperature excess of $150°C$. This curing cycle is not recommended because it is likely to cause likely to cause gaseous porosity.

2) Micro wave:

This is a specially designed electrical computerized device acrylic for curing. In this technique special fiber glass reinforced polyester flasks are used for packing. It has an advantage of saving time as compared to hot water bath.

3) Light cure:

This is used for those acrylics which comprises Urethane diMMA. Visible light is an activator whereas Camphoroquinone serves as an initiator for polymerization.

4) Injection Moulding:

This technique is a continuous pressure injection technique and claims to totally compensate for polymerization and thermal shrinkage that occurs in a heat cured acrylic base.

POLYMERIZATION SHRINKAGE:

Heat activated materials are used in fabrication of nearly all denture bases. Thermal energy required for polymerization of such material may be provided by using a hot water bath, micro wave oven or a light curing unit.

Acrylic has limitation of its final contraction during processing / curing producing volumetric and linear shrinkage. This is because of intermolecular forces (H bonds, Van der Waal's forces etc) in monomer that have to be overcome to allow monomer molecules to add to growing polymer chains. These intermolecular forces maintain monomer molecules relatively far apart in monomer, compared with the structure of polymer. The effect is manifested in comparative densities of monomer and polymer, e.g. for PMMA, density g/cc

Monomer: 0.94   Polymers 1.19

Thus polymer contains more material in less volume. On consideration of these values, it can be shown that volume contraction is approximately 21% for PMMA. In case of dough processing technique, where a ratio of 3:1 w/w polymer is used, a volume contraction of 7% may be expected [1,2,3]. The consequence of this contraction is that, if sufficient dough is used to just fill a mould of desired shape, subsequent polymerization of monomer will cause the material to contract and yield a volume reduction on hardening. Effect is termed CONTRACTION POROSITY[1,2,3].

Contraction porosity is avoided by packing an excess of dough into the mould to allow for contraction .The excess is accommodated through elastic deformation of mould material, where halves of mould are closed under spring pressure

EFFECTS OF SHRINKAGE:

This shrinkage is responsible for derangement of occlusion which if left unadjusted lead to some sore spots on the ridge, lack of proper fit and uneven settling of dentures. According to Wolfaard et al [14, 20] there are many factors that can influence dimensional change of acrylic resin dentures. Where as Wesley et al. [13] found that there are two main factors in production of occlusal discrepancies in processed denture:

i) Change in relationship of teeth or tooth to master cast during processing procedures.

ii) Warpage of denture base through release of inherent strains. When denture is separated from the cast upon which it was processed, tooth may change its relationship to master cast as a result of investing procedures (exothermic reaction of investing stone causing an expansion of wax), careless packing of acrylic resin in moulds or improper closure of flask halves.

Changes in vertical relationships of artificial posterior teeth away from processing cast will be manifested by a space between incisal pin and incisal guide table. If teeth all shift an equal distance in an direction that would increase occluso vertical dimension, the contacts would occur more frequently on more posterior teeth. Heavy contacts on four premolar teeth would be result of one or more of three things.

a) Premolars being displaced farther away from denture base than Molars.

b) Molars, being displaced or intruded toward tissue surface of denture or

c) A lateral shift of one or more of premolars if they are cusped or anatomic teeth.

A lateral shift of any tooth could cause a deflective contact of inclined planes on occlusal surface of opposing teeth which would cause a vertical separation of teeth.

In addition to the factors described by Wesley et al [6] some other workers [7, 9, 11, 12, 19] found other factors which also effect movement of artificial teeth. They are storage of wax pattern, effect of time and temperature, investment procedure/ flasking and packing, type acrylic, maxillary anatomical configurations, denture thickness, processing, cooling and finishing polishing.

First Attiyah [10] then Vieira DF [9] studied the changes in the relative position of teeth during construction of denture bases. They found that original position of teeth during construction of bases is often changed resulting in modification of previously established occlusion. They concluded that wax pattern should not be stored and polymerized as soon as possible.

Ida.M.Harman and Pittsburgh [21] in 1949 found that the linear shrinkage of 0.1% occurs due to time and temperature change.

Perlowiski [18] studied the possibility of investing procedures to cause tooth movement. He investigated by measuring the amount of articulator opening at incisal guide pin after remounting the polymerized denture base.

Grant [11] found that packing and curing also contribute to tooth movement. He concluded that the first pour of investment does not affect the relative position to the cast. The second pour affects the relative positions of teeth on the cast. Tooth movement occurring at this stage, is caused by setting expansion of gypsum and not by thermal expansion of wax produced by heat liberated from setting reaction of plaster. In order to minimize this movement he described a method by clamping the halves of flask upon completion of second pour of the investment.

Dimensional changes that occur at posterior palatal seal of maxillary denture indicates that height of palate may have an influence on amount of distortion that occurs [6]. The internal stresses that developed in acrylic resin dentures during polymerization and are released cause dimensional changes after deflasking and decasting and during and finishing of denture.

Anderson [2, 6] stated that "denture fabricated for bulbous maxillary ridge, will have greater stresses on cooling than a bulky denture for a flat mandibular ridge".

Molligoda [6] studied this phenomenon on clinical casts which were radio graphed and then digitized. Significant correlation was found between palatal form and tooth movement, measured before processing and after deflasking of denture. In the dentures with shallow palates, acrylic shrinkage occurred almost parallel to flat palate and after cooling and deflasking, the stress released pulled the opposing teeth together. Whereas in, dentures with deep palates, thermal shrinkage occurred at an angle along the palatal slopes. After deflasking, release of stresses caused denture to be pulled away from the cast.

Glazier et al [22] reported that palatal base distortion is greater with an increase in palatal height. The distortion caused by denture as it was pulled away from palatal base of cast may have caused teeth to move outwards (buccally). This outward movement of teeth may outweigh the actual linear shrinkage that occurs to pull the teeth together. Thus denture constructed for deep or relatively shallow palates requires more occlusal adjustment during insertion. They also mentioned the role of the maxillary tuberosities and its influence on distortion of the denture base.

Movement of teeth that may occur during finishing and polishing of all of dentures may be caused in part by heat related warpage that may occur during denture trimming, this heat related warpage could also be due to absorption and expansion of denture during trimming and polishing. Similarly Wolef et al [12] measured linear changes across the second molar and buccal flange areas with a tool maker's microscope. They found that greatest changes occurred immediately after deflasking.

Robert G Vig [3, 4] noticed a consistent change in posterior teeth relationship after curing. This problem arises when anterior shift of the maxillary posterior teeth occurs in relation to mandibular posterior teeth. This can always be noted after remounting dentures in which cusped teeth are used. This movement deranges the occlusion in relation to setup in wax; the cusp – fossa relation changes to cusp- cuspal inclines.

A further observation [3, 4] led to a theory that the shift occurred in maxillary denture. When a maxillary denture is first inserted in patient's mouth, disclosing paste demonstrate a derangement of rugae pattern, excessive contact in anterior palatal area and heavy contact of denture against the posterior slopes of the tuberosities. This indicates the shrinkage occurring in forward direction in the maxillary denture base where as no such phenomenon was noted in the mandibular denture. These observations can be explained by the theory that in each instance the labial position of the maxillary alveolar ridge anchored the anterior part of the polymerizing and shrinking resin. So all volumetric and linear contraction occurs in posterior region that causes the movement of teeth in forward direction.

METHODS TO REDUCE SHRINKAGE:

Research [1-3] indicates the polymerization of MMA to form PMMA yields 21% decrease in volume of material. To minimize dimensional changes resin manufacturers prepolymerize a significant fraction of denture base material. This may be thought as "Preshrinking" the selected resins fraction. The prepolymerized material may be mixed with compatible monomer and the resultant mass is then polymerized [1-3].

The accepted polymer monomer ratio is 3:1 by volume. This provides sufficient monomer to thoroughly wet polymer particles. But it does not contribute excess monomer that would lead to increased polymerization shrinkage. Using 3:1 ratio shrinkage may be limited to approximate 6% [1]. Processing changes occur during curing result the overall contraction. In order to minimize contraction different researchers used several curing methods or techniques.

Kenneth [15] in 1964 published an article in which he mentioned movement of teeth due to mishandling during every step of processing. He suggested a method involving a precise step by step technique with particular emphasis on:

    i) Investing in artificial stone.

    ii) Packing only one denture at a time with only mix of acrylic.

    iii) Using minimum pressure while packing with maximum flow time.

    iv) Trial packing until no flash is evident.

Though the method is time consuming but there was less or virtually "no movement" in using conventional method of curing.

Similarly Villa AH [10] described a method which was named as "double processing" technique. This required a special flask. First base was processed to the cast then the processed base was recovered from plaster block without breakage. To avoid an increase in occluso vertical dimension the upper denture base was processed first and occlusion was then corrected against the lower in wax. The lower denture was processed by same technique. No significant movement of teeth was noted.

Recently the induction of Injection Moulding system for curing has claimed to totally compensate for polymerization and thermal shrinkage.

Shermain Salim [14] found that specimen cured by Injection Moulding technique exhibited less dimensional shrinkage then cured by either conventional or Microwave method.

Same study conducted by Keen, Pal [8] also revealed the same results, that injection moulding resulted in a slightly less increases in vertical dimension then conventional method of polymerization.

Robert .G Vig [3, 4] in 1972 keenly studied this polymerization shrinkage myth. By noticing that shift deranges the intercuspation as set up in wax, maxillary cusps tips will contact posterior facing planes of mandibular cusps. He concluded that the shift occurs only in maxillary denture while no such movement in mandibular denture. This difference mainly is due to labial position of maxillary alveolar ridge anchored the anterior part of polymerizing and shrinking resin. So that all volumetric and linear contraction began posteriorly and moved anteriorly, thus carrying posterior teeth forward. In order to test this hypothesis, he mounted edentulous maxillary and mandibular casts on Hanau articulator using mounting jigs. Bases were waxed up and pointed pins were set in maxillary and mandibular ridge areas to exactly oppose each other. The mandibular denture was processed. The pins were still in apposition. Maxillary bases were processed next and pins in maxillary base were found to have moved anterior to mandibular pins. He then substituted the pins with 3mm thick aluminum plates. They were machined to produce interdigitating toothed members. He repeated all the procedures and both pins and aluminum plates gave similar results. However, this investigation did not test possible lateral contraction phenomena. To overcome this problem, an artificial double thickness wax flap was waxed onto posterior of cast. A test case was processed, no shift was observed and articulation remained perfect. This meant that there was practically no pin opening observable at remounting.

To confirm his results Vig asked twenty sophomore dental students to wax corrective posterior flaps onto there upper dentures bases. The rest of class acted as controls. After processing, the twenty experimental cases required little or no grinding, while the control group spent usual two hours, ending up in weird looking teeth.

MATERIALS AND METHODS:

This study was carried out at de'Montmorency College of dentistry /Punjab Dental Hospital, Lahore and PCSIR laboratory Lahore.

Ten maxillary and one mandibular denture were made. The sampling technique was random.

Maxillary dentures were divided in Group A and B. Group A contained the dentures which were to be processed by Conventional curing method while Group B was processed with Vig's technique.

EXPERIMENTAL PROCEDURE:

Cast making and articulation:

In this study ten maxillary and one mandibular denture were prepared. The casts of the dentures were poured in corresponding prototype moulds. They were waxed up with single sheet of dental wax and occlusal rims; measuring 10-12 mm x 5-8 mm in anterior region and 10-12 mm x 7-10 mm in posterior region were constructed. For mandibular base dimensions of the rims were 7-9 x 7-9 mm. Using Bonwill's triangle method, casts were articulated in class I occlusal relationship on Hanau University semi adjustable articulator*. Biometric guide lines were used to set teeth on the rims. Incisive papilla and vestige of gingival margin were taken as a point of reference. They are explained as under:

The posterior aspect of Incisive papilla was taken as reference point in setting of anterior maxillary teeth while receded gingival margin was taken for posterior teeth.

The distance between posterior aspect of incisive papilla and buccal surfaces of Incisors and Canines were 8 mm and 10 mm respectively.

For posterior maxillary teeth the distance was 10mm and 12mm from vestige of gingival margin to buccal cusps.

The centre of the ridge was followed for mandibular set up.

Then mandibular denture was processed which severed as base line for other remaining maxillary set ups.

FORMATION OF JIG FOR MAXILLARY SET UP:

A jig was formed by applying extra hard plaster around buccal surfaces of right side of maxillary teeth in the wax up. After final setting of plaster, same procedure was repeated on left side. Plaster was applied on the palatal side of the teeth in two segments as well.

The remaining nine set ups were performed by using this jig and mandibular denture to make sure that all the set ups were identical.

MEASUREMENT PROCEDURE:

These measurements were recorded according to two indigenous techniques i.e. Manual and Photo imaging.

To measure the movements the reference points were placed on the upper cast and in the artificial teeth.

Manual technique:

On both sides of the base, reference points were selected to measure the superoinferior movement of canine, bicuspids, molars, as shown in Figure B.

For Mesiodistal, Buccopalatal and superoinferior movements of posterior teeth and canines reference points in the form of Amalgam fillings were placed in the mesiobuccal cusp of molars, buccal cusps of premolars, tip of canines and mid point on the incisal edges of incisors.

Holes were drilled with number 2 acrylic trimmer in centre of incisal edges of anterior teeth and buccal cusps of posterior teeth. Amalgam was packed in these holes to act as reference Points. 25 such reference points were inserted in each maxillary set up.

25 individual measurements were taken on each denture according to Figures A and B. These measurements are as follows:

A= bimolar (7 to 7)

B= bimolar (6 to 6)

C= inter premolar (5 to 5)

D= inter premolar (4 to 4)

E= intercanine (3 to 3)

F= right canine to right central incisor (13 to 11)

G= right 1st premolar to canine (14 to 13)

H = right 1st premolar to 2nd premolar (14 to 15)

I=right 2nd premolar to 1st molar (15 to 16)

J= right 1st molar to 2nd molar (16 to 17)

F1= left canine to left central incisor (23 to 21)

G1= left 1st premolar to canine (24 to 23)

H1= left 1st premolar to 2nd premolar (24 to 25)

I1=left 2nd premolar to 1st molar (25 to 26)

J1= left 1st molar to 2nd molar (26 to 27)

On right side:

R1= from reference line to mesiobuccal cusp of 2nd molar.

R2 = from reference line to mesiobucal cusp of 1st molar

R3 =from reference line to buccal cusp of 2nd premolar.

R4=from reference line to buccal cusp of 1st premolar

R5= from reference line to tip of canine.

On left side:

Ll= from reference line to mesiobuccal cusp of 2nd molar .

L2 = from reference line to mesiobucal cusp of 1st molar

L3 =from reference line to buccal cusp of 2nd premolar.

L4=from reference line to buccal cusp of 1st premolar

L5= from reference line to tip of canine.

Measurements were taken at wax up stage and after processing with respect to these reference points. Difference in initial and final readings were calculated on each respective position as shown in figure.

Photo imaging Technique:

Results were verified by Photo Imaging technique.

1) At wax up stage, respective positions as shown in fig A were measured and recorded with respect to their reference points and later on transparencies template were made by photo imaging technique.

2) After curing (method given in section.) the measurements were retaken according to the respective position as mentioned in Figures A, B. These measurements were recorded and template was again made in the final stage under the same magnification as utilized in wax up stage.

3) Both transparencies were superimposed to measure the movement.

GROUPING:

Maxillary set ups were divided into two groups; A and B, each having 5 set ups. The casts in group A were processed conventionally and in group B, using Vig's technique.

VIG'S TECHNIQUE:

It requires an anchorage from the cast to avoid shifting of teeth during curing. To gain this anchorage, posterior aspect of the cast was scrapped to a depth of 0.5 mm approximately. Length and width of the scrapped area was 3.5 x 1 cm. Double wax sheet was used for wax up of this area. The peripheries were properly sealed and dentures were processed.

Flasking was performed using same brand of plaster of Paris. Undercuts were carefully removed. After final set of plaster in 30 minutes, two coats of cold mould seal (sodium alginate) were applied and flasking was completed. Dewaxing was done by placing flasks in warm water for 15 minutes. Trial packing was done after dewaxing for packing of acrylic resins.

Initially curing was to be performed in curing tank using long curing cycle. Failure to use curing tank was for being out of order. Then curing was done in hot water bath.

Flasks were placed in container having water at room temperature. Water was made to boil slowly in two and a half hours. Then flasks were left in boiling water for another half an hour. They were removed after over night cooling in the same water. The cured dentures were removed from the flasks and finished in such a manner that they could be reseated over articulated casts.

Statistical analysis:

A statistical software pack SSPS version 10 for Windows was used to calculate mean standard deviation .For intra group comparison "paired t" was applied. Similarly for inter group "independent t" test was applied.

RESULTS

10 maxillary complete dentures were cured. They were divided into two groups 5 for each group, Vig's and Conventional curing method. One mandibular denture was processed for correct occlusovertical dimension.

The readings were recorded for 25 reference points as shown in fig 1 and 2, before and after curing for both Vig's and conventional method.

A= distance from mesiobuccal cusp of right 2nd molar to mesiobuccal cusp of left 2nd molar (7 to 7)

B= distance from mesiobuccal cusp of right 2nd molar to mesiobuccal cusp of left 2nd molar (6 to 6)

C= distance from buccal cusp of right 2nd premolar to left 2nd premolar (5 to 5)

D= distance from buccal cusp of right 1st premolar to buccal cusp of left 1st premolar (4 to 4)

E= distance between tips of right and left Canine (3 to 3)

On right side:

F=distance between tip of right canine to middle of right central incisor (13 to 11)

G=distance between buccal cusp of right 1st premolar to tip of right canine (14 to 13)

H = distance between buccal cusp of right 1st premolar to buccal cusp of right 2nd premolar (14 to 15)

I= distance between buccal cusp of right 2nd premolar to mesiobuccal cusp of right 1st molar (15 to 16)

J= distance between mesiobuccal cusp of right 1st molar to mesiobuccal cusp of right 2nd molar (16 to 17)

R1= from reference line to mesiobuccal cusp of right 2nd molar.

R2 = from reference line to mesiobuccal cusp of right 1st molar

R3 =from reference line to buccal cusp of right 2nd premolar.

R4=from reference line to buccal cusp of right 1st premolar

R5= from reference line to tip of right canine.

On left side:

F1=distance between tip of left canine to centre of left central incisor (23 to 21)

G1= buccal cusp of left 1st premolar to tip of canine (24 to 23)

H1= buccal cusp of left 1st premolar to buccal cusp of 2nd premolar (24 to 25)

I1=buccal cusp of left 2nd premolar to mesiobuccal cusp of 1st molar (25 to 26)

J1= mesiobuccal cusp of left 1st molar to mesiobuccal cusp of 2nd molar (26 to 27)

Ll= from reference line to mesiobuccal cusp of left 2nd molar .

L2 = from reference line to mesiobucal cusp of left 1st molar

L3 =from reference line to buccal cusp of left 2nd premolar.

L4=from reference line to buccal cusp of left 1st premolar

L5= from reference line to tip of left canine.

TABLE 1(a)

GROUP A

MEAN VALUES AT WAX UP STAGE AND AFTER CURING IN CONVENTIONAL METHOD

Horizontal axis	WAXUP STAGE MEAN(mm) ±STD.	AFTER CURING MEAN(mm) ±STD.	P VALUE
A=Bimolar (7 to 7)	59.56±.699	58.52±.657	.001 S
B=Bimolar (6 to 6)	52.02±1.217	51.560±1.016	.299 NS
C = Interpremolar (5 to 5)	49.460±.351	48.420±.356	.000 S
D= Interpremolar (4 to 4)	42.480±.432	41.400±.412	.006 S
E = Intercanine (3 to 3)	33.160±.134	33.100±.173	.070 NS

TABLE 1(b)

GROUP A

MEAN VALUES AT WAX UP STAGE AND AFTER CURING IN CONVENTIONAL METHOD

ON RIGHT SIDE:

	WAX UP STAGE MEAN (mm) ±STD.	AFTER CURING MEAN (mm) ±STD.	P VALUE
F= Right canine to right central incisor(13 to 11)	15.14±.114	15.100±.141	.178 NS
G =Right 1st premolar to right canine (14 to 13)	8.040±.856	8.12±.164	.855 NS
H= Right 1st premolar to right 2nd premolar(14 to 15)	6.90±.122	7.22±.217	.016 S
I=right 2nd premolar to right first molar(15 to 16)	6.74±.305	6.76±.241	.847 NS
J = right first molar to right 2nd molar (16 to 17)	10.36±.219	9.46±.251	.005 S
R1 = from reference line to mesiobuccal cusp of right 2nd molar	29.30±.212	30.12±.217	.003 S
R2 = from reference line to mesiobuccal cusp of right 1st molar	29.28±.164	30.12±.110	.000 S
R3 = from reference line to buccal cusp of right 2nd premolar	30.00±.000	30.32±.044	.000 S
R4 = from reference line to buccal cusp of right 1st premolar	30.720±.415	31.10±.418	
R5 = from reference line to tip cusp of right canine	31.080±.110	31.08±.110	

TABLE 1(c)

GROUP A

MEAN VALUES AT WAX UP STAGE AND AFTER CURING IN CONVENTIONAL METHOD

ON LEFT SIDE:

	WAX UP STAGE MEAN(mm) ±STD.	AFTER CURING MEAN(mm) ±STD.	P VALUE
F1 = left canine to left central incisor (23 to 21)	15.32 ±.409	15.28±.438	.178 NS
G1 = left 1st premolar to left canine (23 to 24)	8.4±.735	7.64±.371	.012 S
H1 = left 1st premolar 2nd premolar (24 to 25)	7.42±.716	6.84±.428	.012 S
I1 = left 2nd premolar to left 1st molar (25 to 26)	6.100±.000	6.76±.182	.001 S
J1 = left 1st molar to 2nd molar (26 to 27)	10.41±.594	9.88±.249	.246 NS
L1 = from reference line to mesiobuccal cusp of left 2nd molar	33.94±.358	34.80±.447	.000 S
L2 = from reference line to mesiobuccal cusp of left 1st molar	33.98±.110	34.54±.351	.016 NS
L3 = from reference line to buccal cusp of left 2nd premolar	33.500±.464	33.920±.502	.005 S
L4 = from reference line to buccal cusp of left 1st premolar	32.86±.288	33.62±.286	.041 S
L5 = from reference line to tip cusp of left canine	32.78±.179	32.76±.241	.621 NS

TABLE 2(a)

GROUP B

MEAN VALUES AT WAX UP STAGE AND AFTER CURING IN VIG'S METHOD

	WAXUP STAGE MEAN±STANDARD DEVIATION	AFTER CURING MEAN±STANDARD DEVIATION	P VALUE
A=Bimolar (7 to 7)	59.760±.152	59.66±.195	.089 NS
B=Bimolar (6 to 6)	52.100±.574	52.06±.291	.477 NS
C = Interpremolar (5 to 5)	49.24±.241	49.24±.152	1.00 NS
D= Interpremolar (4 to 4)	42.98±.606	42.92±.275	.788 NS
E = Intercanine(3 to 3)	33.900±.000	33.74±.358	.374 NS

TABLE 2(b)

GROUP B

MEAN VALUES AT WAX UP STAGE AND AFTER PROCESSING IN VIG'S METHOD GROUP B

ON RIGHT SIDE:

	WAX UP STAGE MEAN(mm) ±STD.	AFTER CURING MEAN(mm) ±STD.	P VALUE
F= Right canine to right central incisor(13 to 11)	15.200±.0707	15.22±.0447	.374 NS
G =Right 1st premolar to right canine (14 to 13)	8.9±.0707	8.740±.547	.003 S
H= Right 1st premolar to right 2nd premolar(14 to 15)	6.96±.0547	6.92±.130	.374 NS
I=right 2nd premolar to right first molar(15 to 16)	5.72±.217	5.64±.428	.700 NS
J = right first molar to right 2nd molar (16 to 17)	10.560 ±.219	10.40±.235	.306 NS
R1 = from reference line to mesiobuccal cusp of right 2nd molar	29.28±.277	29.42±.311	.025 S
R2 = from reference line to mesiobuccal cusp of right 1st molar	29.26±.251	29.300±.158	.688 NS
R3 = from reference line to buccal cusp of right 2nd premolar	29.86±.434	29.920±.409	.070 NS
R4 = from reference line to buccal cusp of right 1st premolar	30.140±.680	30.200±.700	
R5 = from reference line to tip cusp of right canine	30.840±.416	30.84.416	

TABLE 2(c)

GROUP B

MEAN VALUES AT WAX UP STAGE AND AFTER CURING IN VIG'S METHOD GROUP B

ON LEFT SIDE:

	WAXUP STAGE MEAN(mm) ±STD.	AFTER CURING MEAN(mm) ±STD.	P VALUE
F1 = left canine to left central incisor (23 to 21)	15.840±.134	15.840±.134	.374 NS
G1 = left 1st premolar to left canine (23 to 24)	9.420±.683	9.46±.709	.941 NS
H1 = left 1st premolar 2nd premolar (24 to 25)	6.900±.187	6.840±.219	.749 NS
I1 = left 2nd premolar to left 1st molar (25 to 26)	5.820±.130	5.68±.179	.206 NS
J1 = left 1st molar to 2nd molar (26 to 27)	11.00±.0100	10.78±.444	.374 NS
L1 = from reference line to mesiobuccal cusp of left 2nd molar	34.100±.490	34.24±.518	.005 S
L2 = from reference line to mesiobuccal cusp of left 1st molar	34.22±.327	34.400±.339	.009 S
L3 = from reference line to buccal cusp of left 2nd premolar	33.66±.410	33.82±.349	.016 S
L4 = from reference line to buccal cusp of left 1st premolar	33.04±.747	33.28±.691	.080 NS
L5 = from reference line to tip cusp of left canine	33.800±.714	33.80±.714	

TABLE 3(a)

P VALUE COMPARISON BETWEEN CONVENTIONNAL AND VIG'S CURING METHOD AFTER PROCESSING

	VIG'S METHOD P VALUE	CONVENTIONAL METHOD P VALUE
A=Bimolar (7 to 7)	.089 NS	.001 S
B=Bimolar (6 to 6)	.477 NS	.299 NS
C = Interpremolar (5 to 5)	1.00 NS	.000 S
D= Interpremolar (4 to 4)	.788 NS	.006 S
E = Intercanine(3 to 3)	.374 NS	.070 NS

TABLE 3(b)

P VALUE COMPARISON BETWEEN CONVENTIONAL AND VIG'S CURING METHOD AFTER PROCESSING

ON RIGHT SIDE:

	VIG'S METHOD P VALUE	CONVENTIONAL METHOD P VALUE
F= Right canine to right central incisor(13 to 11)	.374 NS	.178 NS
G =Right 1st premolar to right canine (14 to 13)	.003 S	.855 NS
H= Right 1st premolar to right 2nd premolar(14 to 15)	.374 NS	.016 S
I=right 2nd premolar to right first molar(15 to 16)	.700 NS	.847 NS
J = right first molar to right 2nd molar (16 to 17)	.306 NS	.005 S
R1 = from reference line to mesiobuccal cusp of right 2nd molar	.025 S	.003 S
R2 = from reference line to mesiobuccal cusp of right 1st molar	.688 NS	.000 S
R3 = from reference line to buccal cusp of right 2nd premolar	.070 NS	.000 S
R4= from reference line to buccal cusp of right 1st premolar	.070 NS	.000 S
R5 = from reference line to tip cusp of right canine	.070 NS	.000S

TABLE 3(c)

P VALUE COMPARISON BETWEEN CONVENTIONAL AND VIG'S CURING METHOD AFTER PROCESSING.

ON LEFT SIDE:

	VIG'S METHOD P VALUE	CONVENTIONAL METHOD P VALUE
F1 = left canine to left central incisor (23 to 21)	.374 NS	.178 NS
G1 = left 1st premolar to left canine (23 to 24)	.941 NS	.012 S
H1 = left 1st premolar 2nd premolar (24 to 25)	.749 NS	.012 S
I1 = left 2nd premolar to left 1st molar (25 to 26)	.206 NS	.001 S
J1 = left 1st molar to 2nd molar (26 to 27)	.374 NS	.246 NS
L1 = from reference line to mesiobuccal cusp of left 2nd molar	.005 S	.000 S
L2 = from reference line to mesiobuccal cusp of left 1st molar	.009 S	.016 NS
L3 = from reference line to buccal cusp of left 2nd premolar	.016 S	.005 S
L4 = from reference line to buccal cusp of left 1st premolar	.080 NS	.041 S
L5 = from reference line to tip cusp of left canine	.080 NS	.621 NS

DISCUSSION:

Acrylic resin is a universal choice of material for making complete dentures. During processing, dimensional changes occur but the final contraction is responsible for the derangement of occlusion.

Many factors have been identified for this movement e.g. storage of wax pattern, investment procedures, flasking, packing, anatomy of palate and tuberosities, denture thickness and finishing polishing. To prevent this movement many methods have been devised different workers where as Vig (1972) used a simple posterior anchorage on cast.

For this study ten maxillary complete dentures were constructed which were divided into 2, five for each, groups A and B.

Readings were recorded at wax up stage and after processing. The results in this study support the hypothesis, which depicts that the movement of prosthetic teeth in maxillary denture base is significantly less in Vig's method as compared to conventional curing method.

In this study the movement of teeth during processing of denture has been studied in three regions i.e. Molars, Premolars and Anterior teeth. These movements were recorded in 3 dimensions as Bucco palatal, Anterio posterior, Upward/downward.

CONVENTIONAL METHOD:

Buccopalatal movement in Molar region:

On the horizontal axis A, B (Table 1(a)) i.e. intramolar region had a mean difference of 0.5 to 1.04 mm in wax up and after curing. This indicates the movement in palatal direction due to contraction of acrylic resins in the palatal region. This was also evident when processed dentures were seated over the cast; a visible a space was present between the denture base and the cast in the posterior region.

Upward / Downward movement in Molar region:

For upward and downward displacement (Table 1b and 1c) it was noticed that both right and left molars (R1, L1) have shown downward movement. This movement is contrary to the results of Wesley et al [13] who emphasized that the heavy contacts on four premolars would be the result of intrusion or tissue ward displacement of the molars.

Anterio posterior movement in Molar region:

The distance between 1st and 2nd molars on both sides (J, J1) was reduced suggesting linear shrinkage leading to anterior shift of posterior teeth (Table 1b, 1c). This was noted after remounting dentures on the articulators. This linear shrinkage changed the cusp fossa relationship into cusp-cuspal incline relation in anterioro posterior direction. As a result, the maxillary cusp tips were contacting posterior facing planes of the mandibular cusps as were in the wax up stage.

Bucco palatal movement in Premolar region:

In premolar region there was a difference of 0.32 to 0.58 mm after curing indicating a palatal shift of premolars as observed by measuring the Interpremolar distance (H, H1), contrary to Wesley et al [13] who noted a buccal shift.

(Table 1b and 1c) The distance between left 1st premolar and 1st molar (I_1) showed significant movement of 0.26mm in mesial direction as compared to the right side (I). When cast was inspected and measured in the tuberosities region it was found that the tuberosities width and ridge width had a difference of approximately 1.40 mm in width (Fig 3). This is in conformity that the anatomical configurations influence on dimensional changes. It also supports the observation made by Anderson [6] stating that denture constructed to bulbous maxillary ridge, will have greater stresses on cooling than a bulky denture for flat mandibular ridge.

Similarly Glazier [22] also mentioned the role of maxillary tuberosities and its role on distortion of the denture base. He stated that this could be due to internal stresses occurring during cooling of acrylic resin causing dimensional changes after flasking, decasting and during finishing of denture. The palatal height may also be a contributing factor.

Therefore the significant difference in I_1 and I is due to the difference anatomical configurations.

Upward / Downward movement in Premolars region:

(Table 1b and 1c) Like molars, the premolars (R3, R4, L3, L4) also showed movement of teeth in downward direction or away from denture bearing area.

The distance between left central incisors to canine and right central incisors to canine (E1, F), there was no significant tooth movement observed in anterio posterior, Buccopalatal directions observed. Similarly no upward and / or down ward movement was noticed in Intercanine region E (Table 1a).

Teeth in L4, L5 region also did not show any movement. This is indicative of that no movement in any direction occurred in the anterior region. This "no movement" in anterior region satisfies the observation that in each instance the labial position of the maxillary alveolar ridge anchored the anterior part of the polymerizing and shrinking resin.

VIG'S METHOD:

In Vig's technique readings were recorded similar to Conventional method in the same three dimensions. (Table 2a, 2b, 2c)

Table 2a shows that no appreciable movement of Premolar and Molar teeth occurred in anterio posterior, bucco palatal direction (A, B, C, and D).

There was slight movement of 0.26 mm in anterior direction seen in G region (Table 2b) which could be due to a "palatal shift" of premolars. Similarly slight downward movement in R1, L1, L2, L3 regions (Table 2b, 2c) was observed which again negates Wesley et al. [13] buccal shift observation.

The Intercanine distance E (Table 2a) showed no significant difference in readings before and after curing of the dentures.

Similarly, F, F1 (Table 2b, 2c) showed no movement on right and left sides.

No upward /downward movement in anterior region, R5, L5 (Table2b, 2c) occurred.

Comparing the results of two employed techniques, it was evident that in posterior region movement of teeth was significantly less in dentures which were cured with Vig's method as compared to Conventional curing method. However, in anterior region in both methods no difference was observed due to labial anchorage.

PHOTO IMAGING TECHNIQUE:

For further confirmation of results photo imaging technique was employed. The limitation of photo imaging technique was that it gave results in only horizontal axis .i.e. anterioposterior and Buccopalatal directions. Movements in upward and / or downward directions could not be recorded in this technique.

For conventional technique it was confirmed that molars and premolars moved in anterior and palatal direction. The results were similar for anterior teeth movement in both Manual and photo imaging methods.

On the contrary, photo imaging for Vig's method showed different results supporting the hypothesis that states " VIG`S CURING technique will produce significantly less movement of teeth than CONVENTIONAL curing technique."

Photo imaging was only employed to confirm the results in horizontal axis.

The limitation during this study was non-availability of digital analyzer, which could have given more accurate readings in all dimensions including upward and / or downward directions.

As mentioned previously that prosthetic teeth movement may occur due to other reasons as storing of wax at wax up stage, and finishing and polishing. These variables have not been observed in this study as it for future work.

CONCLUSION:

Occlusal discrepancies are produced in complete dentures as a result of processing procedures. These must be corrected before giving the prosthesis to the patient.

The purpose of this study was the comparison between two curing methods i.e. Vig's and conventional curing methods.

The results of study reveal that:

1. Posterior teeth showed far less movement when dentures were cured with Vig's as compared to Conventional processing technique.
2. Premolars, showed "palatal shift" rather than "buccal shift" as cited in the literature.
3. Extrusion of molars or movement away from tissues occurs instead of intrusion or tissue ward movement.
4. In anterior region in both the techniques no movement was occurred.

Therefore, it is concluded that to minimize the occlusal disharmony in maxillary denture bases after curing, Vig's processing method should be employed which would not only help in reducing the chairside time in occlusal adjustments but also give good functional results.

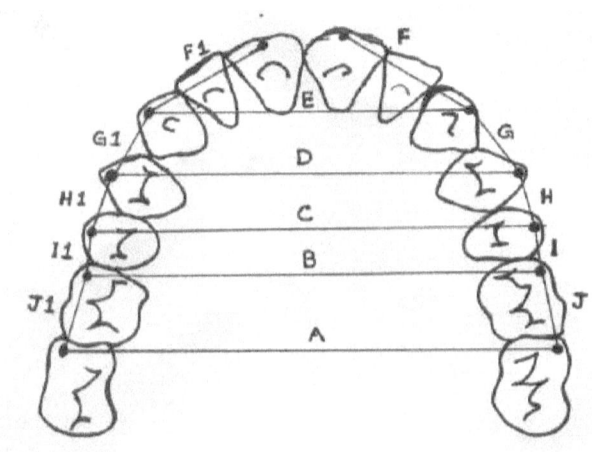

Figure 1: Reference points on teeth measuring the horizontal and anterio posterior movement of teeth

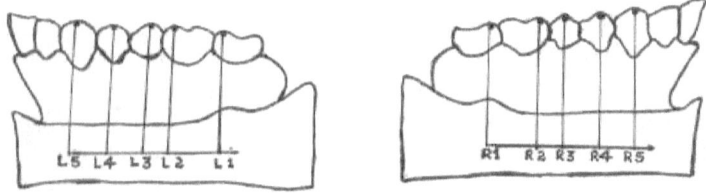

Figure 2: Reference line and occlusal reference points for measuring upward and downward movement of teet

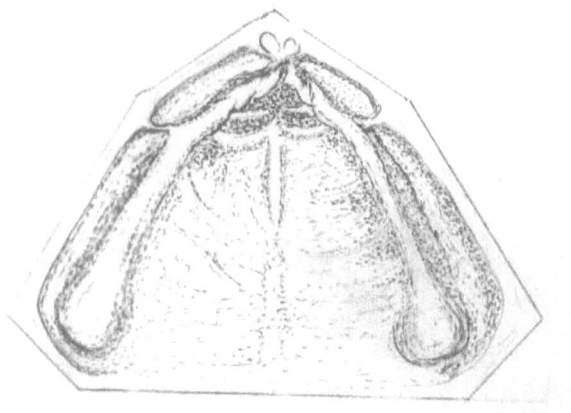

Figure 3: Anatomical configurations of the maxillary cast.

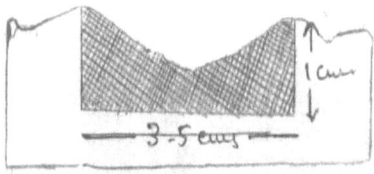

Figure 4: Posterior anchorage in Vig's technique.

REFERENCES:

1. Skinner EW, Phillips RW. The science of dental materials, ed 10th. Philadelphia, W.B Saunders Co., 1996, 242-245.

2. McCabe FJ, Walls WG, Applied dental Materials ed 8th.London, Blackwell Science Ltd; 1998, 96-105.

3. Ray Noel. Dental material science. Lectures: 1999, Wilton; 38-48.

4. Vig RG. Better occlusion and adaptation of dentures, a simple technique 1972

5. Vig RG. Methods of reducing the shift in denture processing. J Prosthet Dent 1975; 33:80-4.

6. Abuzar MAM, Jamani K, Abuzar M. Tooth movement during processing of complete dentures and its relation to the palatal form. J Prosth Dent 1995;73: 445-9.

7. Jamani KD, Abuzar MAM. Effect of denture thickness on tooth movement during processing of complete dentures. J Oral Rehabil 1998;25: 725-9.

8. Keen PL, Radford DR, Clark RK. Dimensional changes in complete dentures fabricated by injection molding and microwave processing .J.Prosth.Dent, 2003; 89: 37-44.

9. Vieira DF, Changes in relative position of teeth in the construction of Denture bases. J.Dent.Res. 1962; 41:1450-60.

10. Villa AH. Double processing technique for complete dentures. J Prosthet Dent 1969; 22:500-5.

11. Grant AA. Effect of the investment procedure on tooth movement, J.Prosth.Dent. 1962; 12: 1053-1058.

12. Lechnar SK, Lautenschlager EP. Processing changes in maxillary complete dentures. J.Prosth.Dent. 1984; 52: 20-24.

13. Wesley RC, Davis H, Quentin Z, Frazier, and Rayson, Processing changes in complete dentures: Posterior tooth contacts and pin opening. J.Prosth.Dent. 1973; 29: 46-53.

14. Salim S, Hamada T. The dimensional accuracy of rectangular acrylic resin specimens cured by three base processing methods. J.Prosth.Dent. 1992 ; 67 : 879-881.

15. Kenneth D. Processing of complete dentures without tooth movement. Dent.Clin.N.Am. 1964; 11: 675-91.

16. Villa H . Double processing technique for complete denture. J.Prosth.Dent. 1969; 10: 500-505.

17. Rueggeberg F A. From vulcanite to vinyl, a history of resins in restorative dentistry. J.Prosth.Dent, 2002; 87: 364-78.

18. Perlowski SA. Investment changes during flasking, a factor of complete dentures malocclusion .J.Prosth.Dent, 1963; 13:269-82

19. Attiyah, AR. Dimensional changes of acrylic resin denture bases influenced by method of processing. Thesis, Northwestern Dental School.

20. Wolfard J, Cleaton J. The influence of processing variables on dimensional changes of heat cured PMMA. J.Prosth.Dent. 1986; 55:518-25.

21. Harman I M, Pittsburg AB. Effects of time and temperature on polymerization of a methylacrylate resin denture base. J.A.D.A. 1949; 38:188-203.

22. Glazier S, Fritell DN, Harman LL. Posterior palatal seal distortion related to height of the maxillary ridge. J.Prosth.Dent. 1980;43:508-10

ANNEXURE

DATA COLLECTION FORM:

DENTURE NO:

WAX UP / AFTER CURING

TECHNIQUE: CONVENTIONAL / VIG'S METHOD

A= bimolar (7 to 7) = _____

B= bimolar (6 to 6) = _____

C= inter premolar (5 to 5) = _____

D= inter premolar (4 to 4) = _____

E= intercanine (3 to 3) = _____

F= right canine to right central incisor (13 to 11) = _____

G= right 1st premolar to canine (14 to 13) = _____

H= right 1st premolar to 2nd premolar (14 to 15) = _____

I= right 2nd premolar to 1st molar (15 to 16) = _____

J= right 1st molar to 2nd molar (16 to 17) = _____

F1= left canine to left central incisor (23 to 21) = _____

G1= left 1st premolar to canine (24 to 23) = _____

H1= left 1st premolar to 2nd premolar (24 to 25) = _____

I1= left 2nd premolar to 1st molar (25 to 26) = _____

J1= left 1st molar to 2nd molar (26 to 27) = _____

On right side:

R1= from reference line to mesiobuccal cusp of 2nd molar. = _____

R2 = from reference line to mesiobuccal cusp of 1st molar = _____

R3 =from reference line to buccal cusp of 2nd premolar. = _____

R4=from reference line to buccal cusp of 1st premolar = _____

R5= from reference line to tip of canine. = _____

On left side:

L1= from reference line to mesiobuccal cusp of 2nd molar. = _____

L2 = from reference line to mesiobucal cusp of 1st molar = _____

L3 =from reference line to buccal cusp of 2nd premolar. = _____

L4=from reference line to buccal cusp of 1st premolar = _____

L5= from reference line to tip of canine. = _____

MATERIALS USED

Monomer (MMA)

Powder (PMMA)

Metro modeling wax

Welbite artifical teeth

 (Medium, H_3 mould)

Dental stone (Hard plaster. Type 2 dental plaster)

Soft plaster (Type 1 Dental plaster)

Cold mould seal (sodium alginate)

Hanau Articulator University model 126.

Amalgam

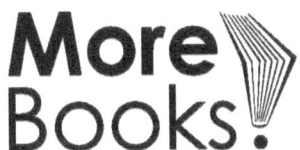

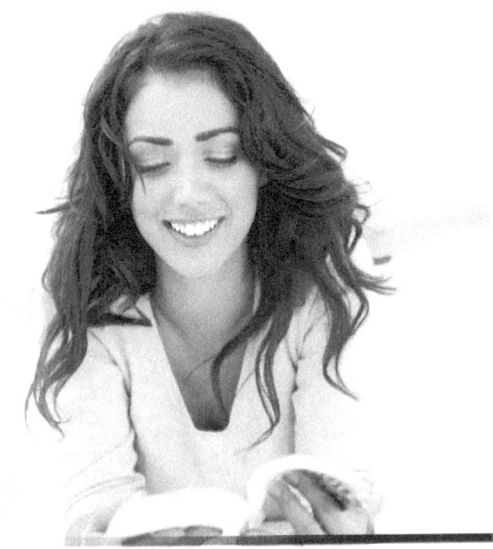

I want morebooks!

Buy your books fast and straightforward online - at one of the world's fastest growing online book stores! Environmentally sound due to Print-on-Demand technologies.

Buy your books online at
www.get-morebooks.com

Kaufen Sie Ihre Bücher schnell und unkompliziert online – auf einer der am schnellsten wachsenden Buchhandelsplattformen weltweit!
Dank Print-On-Demand umwelt- und ressourcenschonend produziert.

Bücher schneller online kaufen
www.morebooks.de

OmniScriptum Marketing DEU GmbH
Bahnhofstr. 28
D - 66111 Saarbrücken
Telefax: +49 681 93 81 567-9

info@omniscriptum.com
www.omniscriptum.com

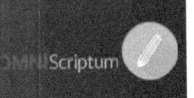

www.ingramcontent.com/pod-product-compliance
Lightning Source LLC
Chambersburg PA
CBHW031541210526
45464CB00003B/1091